I0441680

REAL FOOD & FAKE FOOD:
Over 47 Real food recipes and 10 sure-fire ways to detect fake food!

By Frank Alex

Contents

Introduction

The real question, today is not: are you eating healthy food? But are you eating real or fake food.

You may have given up on junk food, but what about fake food? I'm pretty sure you picture French fries, milk shakes, and potato chips when think about fake foods.

Ironically fake foods are everywhere, they are found lined up on the shelves on the shelves and frozen food sections in most grocery stores, and this includes artificial flavors, popular beverages, preservatives and artificial food colors. These synthetic, food made up of denatured ingredient and petro-chemicals have become a major part of our diets.

Real food is basically food taken directly from nature, without any alterations, or additives.

Most people ultimately end up eating fake food, even though they set out to eat real, healthy food.

Take orange juice as an example. They start with an orange, but then things start going wrong. When was the last time you walked in to a grocery store, to pick up a bottle of orange juice or any other fruit juice for that matter and looked at the ingredient list? Do you see some words on the labels that you can't even pronounce?

Instead of getting some fresh orange or apple juice, the chances are very high that you are consuming a lots of sugar, and preservatives used to maintain freshness

So the foods with additives and artificial colorings become fake, the minute they were processed. Our bodies were made for real food, and these foods found in their natural form, are always better because they are packed with minerals, vitamins, enzymes and a host of other essential nutrients that are helpful in the body.

Our country is the "most obese nation on Planet Earth." Think about this carefully! "2/3rd of Americans are currently obese. "As the saying goes "9 million children under the age of 6 are considered obese."

This means that we are literally destroying our bodies by eating fake foods. It is not so much about or low-fat/no fat, or counting calories, it is about healthy eating today and for the rest of your life.

Sea Food Recipes

Ingredients:

- Toothpicks
- 1 celery stalk, cut into small pcs
- ½ C, plus 2 TBS grated parmesan, divided (optional dairy)
- 1 ½ tsp dried dill • ¼ tsp sea salt • ½ tsp pepper
- 4 TBS melted butter
- 2 cloves garlic, minced • 1 tsp grated lime zest
- ¼ tsp paprika
- ¾ lb sole fillets (or any white fish)
- 1 carrot, peeled and cut into small pcs

Procedure

Preheat oven to 375, then oil a baking dish. Pat the fillets dry and spread them on the baking dish. Place toothpicks in water and let soak...

Mix the butter, lime zest, ½ C parmesan cheese, pepper, garlic, dill, salt, carrot, and celery in a mixing bowl. Divide the mixture into equal portions for as many fillets you have.

Spread the mixture on each fillet, roll the fillet, and secure with toothpick.

Sprinkle the tops of each fillet with paprika and remaining 2 TBS parmesan cheese, then place fillets, rolled side down, in the baking dish.

Bake on the top rack for 30 mins. When done, turn the oven to broil and place the fish under the broiler for 2-3 mins to brown the tops.

Ingredients:

- Sheets of nori seaweed
- Thinly sliced cucumbers
- 1/4 lb (or more) of favorite sliced meat or fish (I've used smoked salmon)
- Avocado
- Thinly sliced carrots
- Any other veggies of choice

Procedure

Break and Whisk one egg, fry it into a thin circle, and use it as the first layer in your roll. Lay the nori shiny side down on a sushi mat.

Lay fried egg down, then place sliced meat on top. Spread avocado over meat in a thin layer or lay slices lengthwise about an inch from the bottom of the nori.

Add a small pile of thinly sliced veggies at the bottom of the nori, too.

Fold the front edge of the nori over the toppings. After each fold, squeeze the roll to secure it tightly, then slice the roll into bite-sized pieces.

Ingredients:

- 1/2 cup almond flour
- 2 TBS of dijon mustard
- 1 egg
- 2 good size pieces of salmon fillets, diced (this can also be used with canned tuna or salmon)
- salt/pepper
- Fresh dill

Procedure

Form the patties and let it settle for 1/2 hrs or longer. Set your pan on med. And place 1 tsp of bacon fat or coconut oil in the pan.

Cook for about 4-5 minutes on each side.

Ingredients:

- 120g Smoked Salmon
- 1 Avocado
- 1 Tbs Olive Oil
- 1 cup Sweet Potato
- 1 Tbs Lime Juice
- 2 Gloves Garlic

Procedure

Boil the sweet potato until it becomes soft. Mash together the avocado and sweet potato, lime juice, olive oil and add finely chopped garlic.

Allow to cool in the refrigerator. Lay out the salmon in strips and place a few spoons of the mash on the salmon.

Roll the salmon up like a sushi roll. Serves one.

Ingredients:

- 1/4 c olive oil
- 1 c sliced almonds
- 1/2 bunch parsley
- 2 shallots
- 1/4 c raisins
- 6 trout
- 2 T olive oil
- 1/2 t pepper
- Lemon, parsley, and seedless red grapes for garnish

Procedure

In a mixing bowl, mix almonds, raisins and olive oil with chopped shallots, parsley and pepper.

Rinse and dry trout and rub body cavity with olive oil. Stuff the trout with this mixture.

Put 1/4 c olive oil in a skillet and sauté each trout for about 8-10 minutes on each side until nicely browned.

Serve with a garnish of lemon, parsley, and seedless red grapes.

Ingredients:

- 1/3 C white wine
- 2 TBS butter or olive oil
- ½ tsp dried dill weed
- 2 - 8 oz fillets of any type of fish
- 1 bunch green onions
- SAUCE
- 2 large cloves garlic, minced
- ¼ tsp sea salt
- 1 TBS Dijon mustard

Procedure

Line a baking pan with foil and coconut oil. Preheat oven to 450. Place fish on pan and arrange onions around fish. Bake in centre of preheated oven until a knife tip inserted into the thickest part of fish and held for 5 seconds comes out warm.

About 7-8 mins. Meanwhile make sauce by placing wine, butter, garlic, dill and salt in a small pan. Bring to a boil over med-high heat.

Boil uncovered and stirring often, until reduced by half, about 2 mins. Whisk in mustard.

Remove fish from pan, spoon garlic-dill sauce over fish and serve onions on the side.

Coconut Shrimp

Ingredients:

- 1 lb. Shrimp
- 2 eggs
- 2 T coconut milk
- 1 tsp curry powder (or more if you want)
- Paprika
- 1 C unsweetened shredded coconut
- Salt and pepper

Procedure

Preheat oven to 350. Beat eggs and coconut milk, set it aside in a shallow bowl, and mix the shredded coconut with a little salt and pepper and curry powder.

One by one dredge shrimp in coconut milk/egg mixture then cover shrimp with shredded coconut mixture.

Put shrimp on oiled cookie sheet (Use coconut oil if you can). Sprinkle with paprika and bake for 20 minutes or until browned.

Ingredients:

- 1/4 c carrots, diced
- 1 t olive oil
- 1 lb small shrimp, peeled and deveined
- 1 t garlic, minced
- 1 t gingerroot, minced
- 8 large iceberg lettuce leaves
- 1/4 c celery, diced
- Toasted pine nuts (optional)

Procedure

In a wok or large nonstick skillet, warm the oil over medium-high heat. Add the shrimp and stir-fry until they are opaque. Remove the shrimp and set aside.

Add the carrots, celery, garlic, and gingerroot to the wok and stir-fry until the vegetables are crisp-tender.

Return the shrimp to the wok and add the wine. Cook until heated through, about 1 minute. Divide the shrimp mixture among the 8 lettuce leaves.

Roll each leaf around the filling and serve. Garnish with the pine nuts, if desired.

Ingredients:

- 1 1/2 t olive oil
- 1t black pepper
- 2 T cilantro or parsley, snipped
- 1 lb sea scallops
- 2 T lime or lemon juice

Procedure

Coat a shallow baking pan with olive oil. Toss scallops with lime juice, cilantro, oil, and pepper.

Arrange scallops in a single layer in pan. Broil until scallops are opaque, 3-4 minutes. Serves 4.

Ingredients:

- 1 TBS of coconut oil
- 1 med onion
- Huge handful of baby spinach
- 1 small jar of green curry paste (Thai kitchen, I believe)
- 2 stalks of celery
- 1 lb of shrimp
- 1 can of coconut milk
- 1 C thinly sliced carrots
- 4-5 sliced mushrooms

Procedure

Heat the coconut oil in a big skillet and set the onions, carrots, mushrooms and celery to browning.

Then add the curry paste and let it fry for a minute until it gets fragrant, followed by the can of coconut milk, and let it simmer for 15 minutes.

Then stir in the spinach until the spinach starts to wilt, followed by the shrimp.

Watch it simmer and remove it from the heat just when the shrimp turns pink. Done!

Meat/Pork Recipes

Ingredients:

- 2 cloves garlic
- 1 stalk celery
- 1 carrot
- 1 small (6 ounce) can tomato paste
- 1/2 c almond flour (or other thickener)
- 1 lb ground beef or turkey
- 1 medium onion
- 1/4 c parsley
- 1/2 red pepper
- 1 egg, slightly beatcn
- Salt and pepper to taste

Procedure

Preheat oven to 375 F. Finely chop the onion, celery, carrot, garlic, parsley, and pepper in a food processor.

In a large bowl, combine all ingredients. Form into a loaf and place in a 9x11 inch glass baking dish coated with oil. Bake for 1 hour. Serves 6.

Ingredients:

- 3 tsp olive oil, divided
- 1 cup ground almonds or other nuts
- 3 Tbs cashew butter
- 1/3 cup egg whites
- 1/2 cup chopped onion
- 2 cloves minced garlic
- 1 chopped red pepper
- 1/2 cup halved grape tomatoes
- 1 large Italian sausage, cut in 1/2" slices
- 1/2 cup marinara sauce (or crushed tomatoes)
- 1/2 tsp oregano
- 1/2 tsp fennel seed

Procedure

Mix ground nuts, cashew butter, and egg whites in a small bowl. Grease a pizza baking sheet or similar with 2 tsp of olive oil, then spread the "dough" mixture over it, making a 1/4" thick crust. Preheat the oven to 250 F.

In a skillet, add the remaining olive oil and the sliced sausage. Cook until browned, then remove the sausage to a small bowl. Add the garlic, onions, and red pepper to the skillet. Sauté the veggies lightly, making sure not to let them get too soft.

Cover the dough with the marinara sauce, then add the meat and vegetables, excluding the tomatoes. Add the oregano and fennel seed, then bake for 30 minutes.

Remove from oven, add the halved tomatoes, and serve! Use a large spatula to carefully remove the slices from the pan, as the nutty "dough" won't be as crisp as traditional grain dough. Makes 4 servings.

Ingredients:

- 1 lb ground beef (or turkey etc.)
- 1 large onion finely chopped
- 5 mushrooms finely chopped
- 3 gloves garlic, finely chopped
- 1 can of crushed tomatoes
- 6 dates, pitted and finely chopped
- 1 TBS favorite herb spice
- 1 med size head of cabbage (red or green)

Procedure

Preheat the oven to 350. You will need a large baking dish, or 2 smaller ones. Boil head of cabbage, removing leaves as they become tender. In a mixing bowl, mix all remaining ingredients, except tomatoes, in a mixing bowl.

Take a cabbage leaf (pat dry if need be) and place about 1/3 C of the meat mixture on the leaf, then wrap it up.

Place stuffed cabbage in the baking dish. Repeat steps until all meat mixture is gone. Pour ½ can of tomatoes over them.

They should all be covered with juice. Bake for 30 mins, take out of oven and pour rest of tomatoes over rolls. Bake for another 20-30 mins.

This is made in a 9x13 baking dish... or something close to that.

Ingredients:

- 1 - 1 1/2 lbs of ground beef or turkey
- 1 head of cauliflower
- 6 green onions
- 1/2 onion (chopped)
- 4 large mushrooms (chopped)
- 3 celery (chopped finely)
- 1 carrot (shredded)
- 2 TBS minced garlic
- 1 TBS Montreal Steak Spice (or something like this)
- 1/2 TBS chili powder
- 1/2 TBS cumin
- ¼ C coconut milk
- 3/4 can of crushed tomatoes (540ml)

Procedure

Preheat oven to 350 F.

Brown ground beef in 1/2 TBS of olive oil, drain fat once cooked. Add the onions, celery, carrots, mushrooms, 1TBS of garlic, Montreal Steak Spice and Cumin. Mix well and cook for 5 minutes.

Add crushed tomatoes, cook on stove until it thickens. Simmer until the cauliflower is ready.

While the meat sauce is cooking you can steam the cauliflower until tender.

Drain the Cauliflower and then beat it or blend it in food processor until it is almost pureed. Add the other 1 TBS of garlic, the chili powder and the coconut milk to the food processor while blending.

Put the meat mixture in the baking pan. Spread the cauliflower on top.

Bake at 350 F for 25-30 minutes.

Meatballs

Are you considering, having meatballs for lunch? Here is a recipe for 30 medium or 20 meatballs

Ingredients:

- 1 tsp red pepper flakes
- 2 eggs, whisked
- 1/2 cup almond meal
- 1/4 cup roughly chopped flat leaf parsley
- 1 lb ground beef (or bison or turkey)
- 1 lb sweet Italian sausage
- 2 cloves garlic, minced
- 1 long sprig fresh oregano, minced
- 1 sprig fresh rosemary, minced
- 3 sprigs fresh thyme, minced
- 1/2 small yellow onion, roughly chopped
- 1/4 cup cream (optional)
- A few grinds black pepper
- 1/2 cup finely shredded parmesan (optional)

Procedure

Unwrap the packaging of the Italian sausage. Excluding the bacon fat, mix all of the stated ingredients, together until well combined.

Roll the meatballs into the desired size, with lightly oiled hands. Heat the bacon fat in a sauté pan over medium to medium-high heat.

Add the meatballs, as soon as it becomes hot. Fry for about 5-7 minutes, until the bottom turns brown. Flip the meatballs to opposite side and fry until that side is nicely browned, another 5-7 minutes.

To determine if it is fully cooked on the inside, you will have to cut one.

If not quite done, cover the pan and turn heat to low for a few more minutes or put meatballs in a warm oven while you fry another set.

Indian Stuffed Peppers

Ingredients:

- 12 oz ground beef
- 2 large red and 2 large green peppers
- 1 onion, finely chopped
- 1/2 tsp cayenne pepper
- Salt
- 1 tsp ground cumin
- 5 Tbsp olive oil
- 2 tsp ground coriander
- 1 can (400 g) tomatoes, keep the liquid

Procedure

Pour and heat about 4 Tbsp of oil in a heated frying pan, then fry the onion until it becomes golden.

Add the spices and cook for 2 minutes. Mix in the ground beef and cook well.

Next, add the salt and cook for a minute. Cut the top of each pepper, removing the ribs and seeds inside. Pour the beef mixture into them.

Ingredients:

- 3-4 lb pork loin roast (well-trimmed)
- Sea salt
- Pepper
- 4-6 apples, cored and quartered
- 1/4 c pure apple juice
- 3 T raw honey
- 1 t ginger

Procedure

Rub roast with salt and pepper. Brown under broiler to remove excess fat, then drain well. Place apples in bottom of crock pot. Add roast.

Combine rest of ingredients, spoon over roast. Cook on low 10-12 hours.

Ingredients:

- 1 small apple, diced (I left the skin on)
- 2 small celery stalks, chopped
- 2 T dried cherries, chopped
- 2 T chopped pecans
- 2 T fresh chives, chopped
- 1 T fresh Italian parsley, chopped
- 2 T apple juice or apple cider
- Some ground nutmeg
- 1 lb. pork tenderloin, trimmed of fat
- Sauce: • 1/4- 1/2 cup apple juice or cider (organic 100% juice)
- 1 tsp arrowroot (thickener, and paleo!)
- Dash cinnamon

Procedure

Stir together apple, celery, pecans, chives, parsley and nutmeg. Add a splash (1-2 T apple juice). Butterfly pork loin: make a single lengthwise cut down the center of the roast, cutting within 1/2 inch of the other side.

Spread the meat open. Cover meat with plastic wrap and pound to about 1/2 inch thickness. Spread stuffing over meat.

Roll up from on the short sides and tie with string to secure. Brush pork with a little remaining apple juice from the mixture.

Place meat on a baking dish and, and bake, uncovered for about 1 hour (or until internal temperature reaches 175 degrees).

In a sauce pan, stir together apple juice and arrowroot powder. Cook and stir until thick and bubbly (it doesn't take long). Pour over sliced pork roast.

Vegetable Recipes

Ingredients:

- 1 T olive oil
- 1 large onion, chopped
- 1/2 med head red cabbage, cored and shredded
- 1/4 t freshly ground black pepper
- 1/4 t ground allspice
- 3 med sweet-tart apples (such as Golden Delicious), peeled, cored and cut into thin wedges
- 1/4 c apple juice, frozen concentrate
- 2 T red wine

Procedure

In a large saucepot or Dutch oven, heat the oil over medium heat. Add the onion and cook, stirring frequently, for 6 minutes or until soft. Add the cabbage, pepper, and allspice.

Cook, stirring frequently, for 4 minutes or until the cabbage begins to wilt and the color starts to change.

Add the apples, apple juice concentrate, and wine. Bring to a boil.

Reduce the heat to low, cover, and simmer, stirring frequently, for 15 minutes, or until cabbage is tender.

Ingredients:

- ½ small white onion (optional)
- 2-4 tablespoons butter, room temperature
- 3 broccoli heads, cooked and stems removed
- 1 lb. carrots, cooked well, skinned, and diced small
- Salt and pepper (to taste)

Procedure

Steam the broccoli and carrots. Add broccoli and carrots to the food processor, and blend well. Add onion and puree until it is well mixed.

When onion, broccoli, carrots, are well-blended, transfer to a medium bowl and add 4 TBS of butter and give the mixture a nice blend using a metal spoon or spatula. The butter should melt.

Ingredients:

- 1 small cabbage, cored
- 2 T olive oil
- 1/2-1 t onion powder (optional)
- 1/8-1/4 t black ground pepper
- 4 medium carrots cut into 1-inch pieces
- 2 celery ribs cut into 1- inch pieces
- 1 small onion cut into wedges
- 1/2 lb whole mushrooms
- 1 small green pepper cut into pieces

Procedure

Cut cabbage into 6 wedges; spread oil on cut sides. Place cabbage on a piece of heavy-duty foil, about 24x18 inches. Sprinkle with onion powder, if desired and pepper.

Arrange remaining vegetables around cabbage. Seal the foil tightly.

Grill, covered, over medium-hot heat for 30 minutes or until vegetables are tender, turning occasionally.

Ingredients:

- 1 spaghetti squash
- 1 ½ C broccoli, chopped
- 5-6 mushrooms, sliced
- 1 small onion
- 1 lb ground beef
- 3 eggs
- Half can coconut milk
- Asst. spices/herbs (I used Montreal Steak Spice)
- Handful of slivered almonds

Procedure

Preheat oven to 350. Cut Squash in half lengthwise, and place cut side down in shallow baking dish with a bit of water. Cook for 45 mins. Meanwhile, brown the ground beef and steam the broccoli, just so it softens up a bit.

Sauté the mushrooms and onions with the ground beef. In a mixing bowl, whisk 3 eggs/half can coconut milk/spices+herbs.

Putting it all together: Fork the spaghetti squash out of its shell, so it's in strands. Put the spaghetti squash at the bottom of your baking dish as a first layer.

Then add the ground beef, broccoli, mushrooms, and onions into the egg mix – mix it all up! Pour this over your spaghetti squash.

Throw into oven and bake at 350 for about 40 mins.

Just before it's done, throw some slivered almonds on the top and turn the oven to Broil for a few minutes so that the almonds become toasted.

Ingredients:

- 1 1/2 lb small zucchini, thinly sliced
- 2 T olive oil
- 2 T olive oil
- 1 medium onion, chopped
- 2 apples, chopped
- 2 tomatoes, peeled and chopped
- 2 T chopped parsley
- pepper to taste

Procedure

Set a small pan of water to boil. Drop the zucchini slices into the boiling water for 30 seconds. Remove immediately and drain.

Heat the oil in a fry pan and sauté the onion until it is transparent. Add the apples and stir well to coat.

Add the tomatoes and the blanched zucchini. Stir well, and then add the parsley.

Season this mixture, and leave it to cook, covered over a gentle heat for 5-10 minutes, until the zucchini is soft. Serve hot.

Ingredients:

- 2 or 3 Eggplants
- Olive Oil (lots)
- 1 cup very thinly sliced celery
- 1 onion, chopped fine
- 1 cup tomato sauce (homemade or canned)
- 1/2 cup pitted green olives, roughly chopped
- 3 Tablespoons capers, rinsed and drained
- 2 chopped anchovy fillets (rinsed and drained if packed in salt)
- 1/4 cup red wine vinegar
- 1 Tablespoon honey

Procedure

Preheat oven to 375°F. Remove the stem ends from the eggplant and cut into 1 inch cubes.

Toss the eggplant cubes with 2 tablespoons of olive oil, place on a baking sheet, and roast in the oven until golden (20-30 minutes).

Meanwhile, heat a tablespoon of olive oil in a pot or Dutch oven over medium heat. Add the celery and sauté until it's golden.

Set the celery aside, add another tablespoon of olive oil and the onion and cook for about 10 minutes.

Pour the tomato sauce over the onions, stir, and cook for 10 minutes more.

Add the roasted eggplant, celery, olives, capers, anchovies, vinegar, and honey.

Mix well and cook for 10 minutes more. Taste and adjust for acidity.

Ingredients:

- 4 cups butternut squash, peeled and grated
- 1 small onion, peeled and grated
- 3 eggs, whisked
- Bacon fat, for frying

Procedure

In a large bowl make latke batter by mixing together squash, onion and eggs. Use your hands to form batter into 3 inch patties.

In a large skillet, heat fat, fry patties on each side over medium heat until golden brown and crispy.

Remove latkes from pan and place on a paper towel lined plate to drain excess oil. Repeat Steps 2-4 until batter is used up.

Can be served with applesauce, sour cream or yogurt. (Sometimes the patties don't stay intact, so I actually take a big mound of the mixture and put it in the pan and pat it down flat with my spatula. (This seems to work better).

Ingredients:

- 2 large zucchinis
- 1 lb ground bison/buffalo (or ground turkey or other meat)
- 1/2 large onion, minced
- Salt and pepper to taste
- Dash of cayenne pepper
- 1/2 t of oregano
- 1 8 oz can tomato sauce
- 1 T tomato paste (optional)
- 1/2 c chopped olives or olive tapenade
- 1 egg
- Coconut oil

Procedure

Cut the zucchinis in half (long). Scoop out the insides to form a large trough in each zucchini.

Heat coconut oil in a skillet and sauté the onion and the scraped out zucchini insides. Caramelize it and make sure all the water cooks out.

Remove the zucchini/onion mixture to a large bowl. Add the meat to the skillet and brown, along with some salt and pepper to taste, the cayenne, and the oregano.

Drain it if there is a lot of liquid after the meat is done cooking.

Add the tomato sauce and paste and stir to combine. Add the meat/tomato mixture to the bowl with the onion/zucchini mixture, along with the olives.

Mix well and make sure it is slightly cool. Beat the egg and mix it in.

Mound each zucchini half with the mixture and put in a large baking dish with a little water on the bottom. Bake at 400 F for 40 minutes.

You can make the filling and stuff the zucchinis in advance and hold them covered in the fridge until it is time to bake them. Serves 2.

Kelp noodles are a great substitute for pasta. They are made from nothing but kelp, and are very low carb.

An entire 12 oz package only contains 3g of carbohydrate and totals 18 calories! If you are tired of spaghetti squash, or looking to get a few more trace minerals into your diet, these are the way to go! Quick, easy, and very versatile.

Look for packages of kelp noodles in the refrigerator section of better markets.

Ingredients:

- 1 lb pork, cut into cubes
- 12 oz kelp noodles
- 1/2 cup chopped onions or leeks
- 1 cup chopped celery
- 1 small red bell pepper, seeded and chopped
- 1 Tbsp coconut or olive oil
- 1 Tbsp chopped ginger
- 2 Tbsp Tamari (wheat free) soy sauce
- 2 cloves crushed garlic

- 2 Tbsp arrowroot powder
- Pepper to taste

Procedure

Heat the oil in a large skillet or wok. Add the ginger and the onions (or leeks), sauté 2 minutes. Add the meat, turning often, until browned on all sides. Next, add the remaining vegetables except the garlic. Sauté for 5 minutes, then add the kelp noodles and soy sauce.

After several more minutes, add the arrowroot to thicken the sauce, and the crushed garlic.

Toss well until the sauce has thickened, then serve. Top with fresh ground pepper.

Sautéed Kale

Ingredients:

- 1 lb kale trimmed and chopped
- 1 large garlic clove, crushed
- 1 T olive oil
- 2 T walnuts, lightly toasted
- 2 T lemon juice

Procedure

Cook the kale in a large pot of boiling water until tender (about 10 minutes); drain well. Coat a large skillet with oil. Sauté garlic over medium heat until just golden (about 3 minutes).

Add kale to skillet. Stir in the olive oil, sauté until heated through (about 5 minutes).

Stir in pine nuts, remove skillet from heat. Sprinkle kale mixture with lemon juice. Transfer to a shallow serving dish and serve immediately.

Sautéed Broccoli

Ingredients:

- 1 t olive oil
- 2 or 3 garlic cloves, minced
- 1 onion, diced
- 4 or 5 button mushrooms, thinly sliced
- 1 or 2 tomatoes, diced
- 1 head broccoli, cut into small flowerets, with stems peeled and thinly sliced

Procedure

Bring a large pot of water to boil over high heat. Add broccoli and cook until bright green but not completely tender, about 3 minutes.

Plunge into cold water to stop the cooking process and preserve the bright color.

Heat oil in a skillet over medium heat. Add garlic, onion and cook, stirring for 2-3 minutes. Remove cover and stir in broccoli.

Simmer uncovered for 2-3 minutes.

Eggplant Pizza

Ingredients:

- 1 large sized eggplant
- 1 can pure tomato sauce
- 1 t basil
- 1 t oregano
- Other toppings as desired

Procedure

Slice the eggplant lengthwise, making probably 6-8 slices about 1/2 inch thick. Place on a greased cookie sheet and place under a broiler.

Broil until light brown. Remove, flip and cover with tomato sauce, basil, and oregano.

Feel free to add more toppings – peppers, onions, pepperoni, and diced ham.

Place back under the broiler.

Ingredients:

- 1 TBSP Olive oil
- Garlic Clove
- Heat in pan at med heat for about 2 minutes
- 3 Tbsp. Balsamic Vinegar
- 4 Tbsp. Water
- 1 Tbsp. Butter (optional)
- Parsley

Procedure

Simmer one minute Add Asparagus. Simmer until tender.

Chicken & Turkey Recipes

Stuffed Chicken Breast

Here is a tasty and quick protein recipe. They can be made ahead of time and served for lunches and snacks. You can be creative with seasonings, as you can experiment with your favorite spices, fresh herbs and. I used thyme, oregano, garlic powder for this set.

Ingredients:

- Shredded spinach
- Chopped tomato
- Large boneless, skinless chicken breasts
- 1-2 Tbsp tahini per chicken breast
- Seasonings to taste

Procedure

With a sharp fillet knife, slice the chicken breasts lengthwise, making a pocket to stuff. Spread the tahini in each chicken pocket.

Fill with the spinach and tomato, or other veggies of your choice.

Add any seasonings, close the chicken breast, and place in a baking dish.

Bake in the oven at 350 degrees for 30 minutes.

Ingredients:

- 3.5 lbs. of chicken
- 1 can coconut milk
- 1 sweet onion
- 2 green peppers
- 2 tsp fresh grated ginger
- 2.5 tsp curry
- 2.5 tsp garam marsala
- 1.5 tsp cardamom
- 4 T butter
- 1 can tomato paste
- 1 cup yogurt when finished cooking (optional)

Procedure

Throw it all in the crockpot. Don't even bother to mix it, just throw it in and put it on low for 8 hours. After 8 hours, mix in the yogurt and then stir.

You should have a nice thick, delicious sauce now. I removed the chicken and actually whisked the sauce to make it smooth before putting the chicken back in.

Prep took about 10 minutes. Feel free to add the same amount of curry and grand marsala at the end as well.

Make it stronger. This will make about 5-6 meals depending how much you eat in a sitting. If anything, it makes enough sauce that you could probably toss in another pound or two of chicken no problem.

Next time I'm just going to use a whole chicken and piece it before putting it in the crockpot.

Turkey Stuffed Zucchini

Ingredients:

- 1 zucchini about 12 inches long, or 6 medium ones
- 3 T olive oil
- 1/2 c chopped onion
- 3 cloves garlic minced
- 1/2 c chopped mushrooms
- 2 T dry white wine
- 1 lb ground turkey
- 2 diced tomatoes
- 3 T chopped basil
- 1 t chopped rosemary
- 1 egg, lightly beaten
- 2 t sea salt
- 2 t pepper

Procedure

Cut zucchini in half lengthwise. Scoop out insides, leaving shells about 1/4 inch thick. Reserve about half of the insides.

Heat 2 T of olive oil in a skillet on medium high heat. Sauté onion and garlic until soft.

Add mushrooms and reserved zucchini insides, and sauté another 2 minutes.

Ingredients:

- 2 boneless skinless chicken breasts, sliced into fingers
- 1 egg, beaten
- 1/2 c almond flour
- 1/2 t sea salt
- 1.5 t poultry seasoning
- 1 t dry mustard powder
- 1/4 - 1/3 c olive or coconut oil for frying

Procedure

Heat the oil in a large pan over medium heat.

Place the beaten egg in one bowl and the almond flour plus seasonings into another bowl.

Dip each chicken breast in egg, then in the almond flour mixture.

Cook the chicken in two batches until it is golden on each side.

Luke's Chicken and Spinach

Ingredients:

- 4 Chicken breast cut up into bite size pieces
- 5 big mushrooms, sliced
- 4 small yellow onions, sliced
- 3 cups spinach
- 1 TBS olive oil
- ½ TBS oregano
- ½ TBS herb spice (your choice)
- Handful of raisins
- Handful of almonds
- 1 ripe avocado

Procedure

Pan fry chicken in oil and add the spices. Once chicken is cooked, add the onions and mushrooms and sauté.

Once the mushrooms and onions are browned, add the spinach, raisins and almonds.

Cook for another couple minutes. Top with avocado.

Ingredients:

- 4 large chicken breasts
- ½ C almond flour
- ¼ tsp sea salt
- ¾ tsp dried basil
- ¾ tsp dried oregano
- ½ tsp dried thyme
- 1 ½ tsp olive oil
- 2 large eggs Tomato paste or tomato sauce Asst Pizza toppings: mushrooms, peppers, sausage, bacon, spinach, tomatoes, shrimp, pineapple etc.

Procedure

Preheat oven to 350. Combine all above ingredients in a food processor, except your pizza toppings. Mix well.

Grease a cookie sheet with coconut oil. Spread the chicken mixture from end to end of the cookie sheet with a spatula.

This makes the crust nice and thin. Bake in oven for 15 mins.

Take out crust, spread on tomato sauce then add all your toppings. Put in oven for another 15-20 mins.

Ingredients:

- 3 tablespoons ketchup
- 3 garlic cloves, minced
- 1 large egg
- 3 tablespoons olive oil
- 1 lb. ground organic turkey meat
- 1 small onion, minced

Procedure

Mix together egg, onion, garlic, ketchup, in a medium sized bowl. Mix in turkey meat and mash mixture with hands. When well-mixed, form 1-inch diameter meatballs and set aside on a cookie or baking sheet.

Thoroughly wash your hands before moving on. Heat oil.

Over a medium-heat skillet, transfer meatballs to skillet and cook until brown on all sides when flipped. Drain the excess oil, when cooked, then transfer to plate, and serve.

Chicken with Turmeric

Ingredients:

- 1-2 garlic cloves
- 1 1/3 C chopped onion
- 1 inch piece of fresh ginger
- 1/4 C lemon juice
- 2 Tbsp olive oil
- 1 lb boneless chicken breast
- 1 tsp turmeric

Procedure

Add garlic, 1/3 cup onion, ginger, and lemon juice to a blender. Process to a fine pulp, then set aside. Sauté the remaining onion in a skillet with the olive oil.

Cut chicken into bite-sized pieces, then add to onion and cook, stirring until browned. Add the turmeric and garlic pulp. Cook for 5 minutes, stirring frequently.

Ingredients:

- 1/2 lb ground turkey
- 1 Tbsp olive oil
- 1 cup shredded carrots
- 6 omega 3 eggs
- 5 Tbsp coconut milk
- 1/2 cup beef broth
- 4 Tbsp fresh parsley
- 1/2 tsp coriander
- Coconut oil

Procedure

Brown the turkey in a bit of olive oil in a skillet over medium heat. Meanwhile, shred the carrots. Crack the eggs into a bowl; beat well with a wire whip.

Add the meat when done, carrots, and all of the remaining ingredients except the coconut oil. Stir.

Grease a baking dish or pie pan with some coconut oil. Pour in the mixture, then bake at 250 degrees for 20-30 minutes.

You will need to check on it periodically; it is done when the center is firm and a knife pushed into it comes out clean.

EGG, SOUP & SALAD RECIPES

Daniel's Zucchini Omelet

Ingredients:

- 1 onion
- 1/3 red bell pepper, finely chopped
- 4 mushrooms, thinly sliced
- 3 tsp olive oil
- 1 medium or 2 small zucchini's, grated
- 6 eggs • ½ tsp sea salt
- ½ tsp pepper
- 1 tsp Montréal steak spice (or your favorite herb spice)
- 2 TBS slivered almonds

Procedure

In a stovetop pan (deep sides and has lid), sauté the onion, peppers and mushrooms in 1 tsp of the olive oil for 5-6 mins. Set aside.

Heat the remaining 2 tsp of olive oil over medium heat in the stovetop pan, add the zucchini and brown it.

Once it has lightly browned layer the bottom of the pan with the zucchini and then add the onion mixture. Layer on top of zucchini.

Whisk eggs together in a small bowl, add all the spices. Pour the eggs into the pan. Add the almond slivers.

Cover the pan with a lid and reduce heat to low. The omelet will puff slightly when done.

Apples can be combined with celery to make this fine soup spiced with curry. Get a juicy apple for this recipe.

Ingredients:

- 2 sprigs fresh parsley
- 4 cups diced celery root
- 1 tbsp lemon juice
- 2 tsp curry powder • 4 cups chicken stock
- 1 bay leaf (optional)
- 1/4 tsp crushed dried mint
- 1 tsp sea salt
- 3 tbsp coconut oil
- 1 cup finely chopped leeks (white part only) or onions
- 2 cups peeled, cored chopped apples (about 2)
- 1 sprig dried thyme or 1/4 tsp crushed dried
- 1/4 tsp freshly ground pepper
- 1 cup coconut milk

Procedure

Melt butter over low heat in a large heavy saucepan, then add celery root, leeks and cook until moist, while it's partially covered, for 10 minutes, stirring at intervals.

Mix in curry powder, and apples, then cook for 5 minutes.

Add bay leaf, thyme, stock, parsley, salt and pepper; allow it to boil, turn down the heat and simmer very gently, while still covered, until apples, and celery root are tender, after about 30 to 40 minutes.

Puree soup in food processor or blender and pour into clean saucepan.

Add cream/milk, lemon juice, and mint, then heat through.

Get warmed soup bowls and pour out hot soup into them.

Sprinkle mint and float a lemon slice in each bowl and serve.

Indian Style Slaw

Here is an easy, cheap veggie idea. If you use a bag of readymade broccoli slaw, you can really save time.

Tomatoes are optional. Though this is a stand-alone veggie dish, you could add some leftover meat to this for a complete meal.

Ingredients:

• 1 bag broccoli slaw

• 1 cup fresh diced tomatoes (optional)

• 1 Tbsp olive oil

• 1 tsp mustard seeds

• 1 tsp cumin

• 1/4 tsp turmeric

• 2 Tbsp lemon juice

Procedure

Heat 1 Tbsp of olive oil over medium heat in a skillet, add 1 tsp of mustard seeds. Cover and cook until the seeds stop popping.

Next, add the whole bag of slaw, the tomatoes (if using), plus 1 tsp cumin and 1/4 tsp of turmeric.

Sauté for 3-5 minutes, tossing occasionally, until the slaw is soft.

Add 2 Tbsp of lemon juice. Stir and serve.

Cauliflower Celery Soup

Ingredients:

- 1 large head of cauliflower
- 2-3 celery stalks
- 1 carrot
- 2 cloves garlic
- 1-2 onions
- 1-2 t ground cumin
- 1/2 t pepper
- Parsley springs
- 1/4 t sage

Procedure

Chop head of cauliflower (save a handful of tiny flowerets for a raw garnish) and put in soup pot. Chop and add: celery, carrots, garlic, and onions. Add spices. Barely cover with water, bring to boil and simmer until veggies are tender.

Blend the contents of the pot and adjust seasonings to taste.

Add a little hot water if the soup is too thick. Serve garnished with raw flowerets.

Chicken Apple Salad

Ingredients:

- 6 oz chicken
- 6 cups shredded cabbage
- 1/2 Grannysmith apple
- 1/2 tsp allspice
- 1/8 tsp cloves
- Olive oil
- Sea salt and pepper to taste

Procedure

Dice the chicken. Heat 1 tsp of olive oil in a skillet over medium heat. Add the chicken, allspice, and cloves. Sauté, tossing often, until the chicken is cooked thru.

Shred the cabbage into a large salad bowl. Slice half of an apple into very thin slices and set them aside.

Once the chicken is done, add it to the cabbage, then top with the apple. Add salt and pepper to taste, then drizzle with olive oil.

Use an appropriate quantity of olive oil to meet your individual needs.

Chris' Egg Muffins

Ingredients:

- 1/8 cup water
- 1/4 tsp salt
- 1/2 cup diced vegetables
- 6 eggs
- 1/8 tsp ground pepper
- 1/4 – 1/2 cup cooked meat, cut or crumbled into small pieces

Procedure

Generously grease 6 muffin tins with butter or coconut oil or for easier removal line with paper baking cups, after preheating the oven to 350 degrees .Beat the eggs in a mixing bowl.

Add meat, vegetables, ground pepper, salt, and any other ingredients and stir thoroughly.

Pour into the muffin cups. Continue baking for 18-20 minutes until a knife inserted into the center of a muffin comes out almost clean.

Take away the omelets from the muffin cups and serve.

Ingredients:

- 3 eggs
- 2 Tbs coconut milk
- 1 Tbs honey (I leave it out)
- 2 Tbs melted butter
- 1 Tbs grapeseed oil (or another Tbs of butter, but I like them better with the oil)
- 1/4 tsp salt
- 1/2 tsp baking soda
- 3 Tbs coconut flour

Procedure

I put the batter in the fridge for the butter to solidify (fluffier pancakes) and then cook them however you normally cook pancakes.

I use medium heat and a slightly buttered non-stick pan (the only time I use Teflon anymore). They store great and hold toppings well.

Perfect Hard Boiled Eggs

The secret to making the perfect hard boiled eggs is as follows:

• Fill your pot with water.

• Drop the eggs into the water (make sure the eggs are just covered by the water).

• Add some vinegar (optional, this will help the eggs not crack)

• Stick pot on a hot element – HI.

• Boil for exactly 12 minutes (the yolk will be medium soft – add a minute if you like your yolk hard).

• Remove from stovetop and run cold water into the pot for a minute.

• Let stand for one minute. Drain all water (if you don't drain the water right away, they will become harder to peel). Peel & enjoy!!

When you eat real food your body absorbs nutrients essential for metabolism, which makes glowing skin, weight loss, emotional well-being and overall vitality easier to achieve.

Choosing what to eat is very important, as you are what you eat. How to know real food from fake foods?

Here are a few simple, practical and non-complicated tips that will help you read ingredient labels and identify fake foods:

1. Like my grandma would say, "Keep it simply stupid. I have found that over time that long ingredient lists raise red flags.

2. Be cautious when doing your grocery shopping and look for, labels that tell that the product, is "certified organic, and/or all-natural".

3. Look out for products you are familiar with; You don't want to be ingesting food products if you can't pronounce it or has long chemical names, or picture it while growing up.

4. Download and use the app, Don't Eat That, to get information about the plethora of things that specific food contains.

5. Remember that ingredients are listed according to their proportion in the product. This usually means that the top

three ingredients are in higher proportions, so you are essentially eating those three ingredients.

6. Buying organic, fresh or minimally processed foods, as ingredient listings don't usually list contaminants that the food might have been exposed to, such as solvents and pesticides

7. Usually all flour gotten from wheat is called wheat flour even if it has been bleached and processed. Don't be deceived, go for whole grain flour, as it's a very healthy form of wheat flour.

8. Watch out for food products that are deceptively packaged into small sizes. Manufacturers use this trick on

consumers to reduce the number of essential grams of sugar, fat and calories believed to be in the food.

9. Look out for words like "raw", "sprouted", as they indicate that the food is of a higher quality

10. Don't be deceived into thinking that brown food products are healthier than white food products. For example brown sugar is just white sugar that has been coated with brown coloring and flavoring.

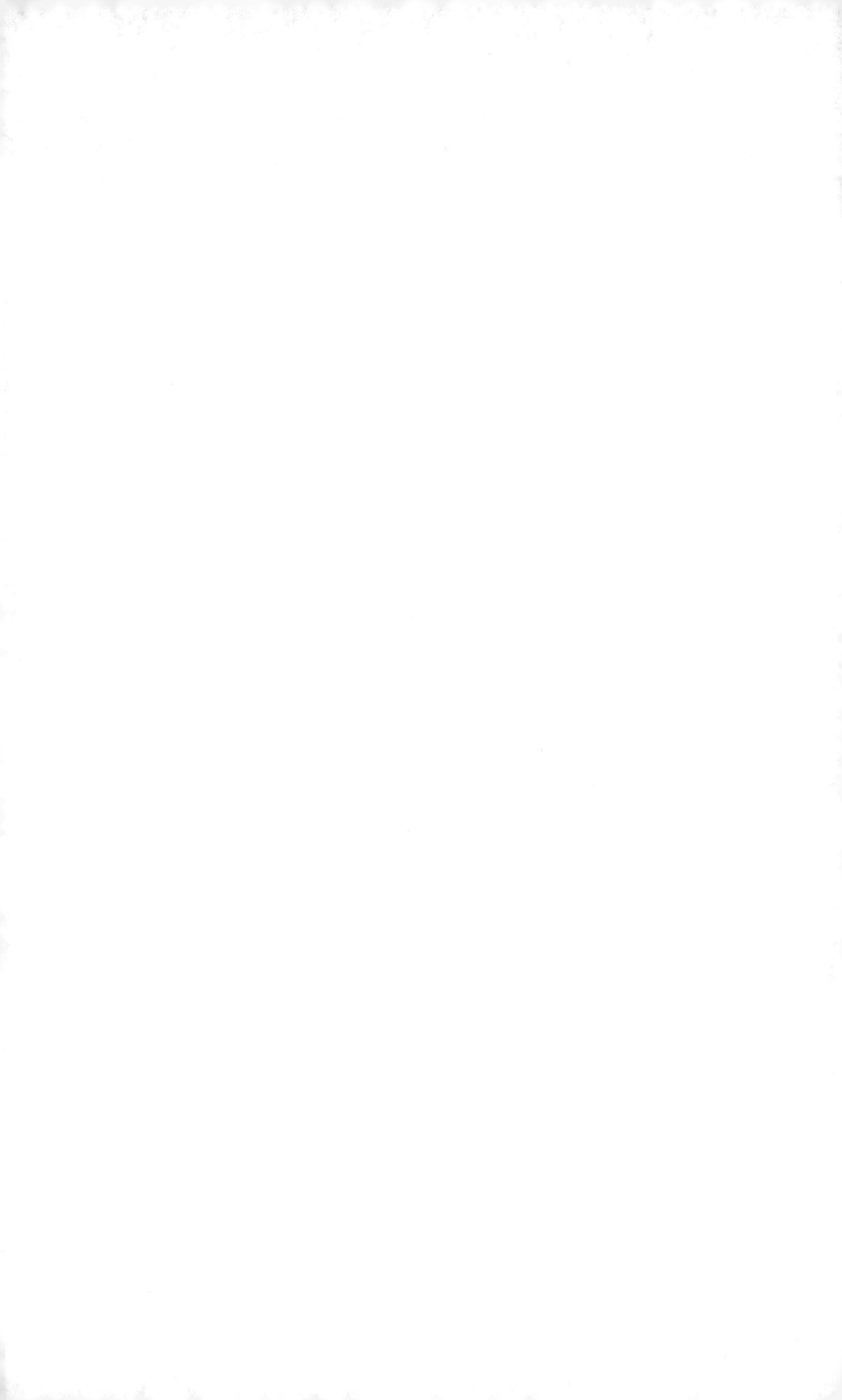

www.ingramcontent.com/pod-product-compliance
Lightning Source LLC
Chambersburg PA
CBHW060639290526
45793CB00001B/323